PAIN MANAGEMENT DECODED

SURVIVING AND THRIVING WITH CHRONIC PAIN

PAIN MANAGEMENT DECODED

Surviving and Thriving with Chronic Pain

By

Dr. JB Kirby

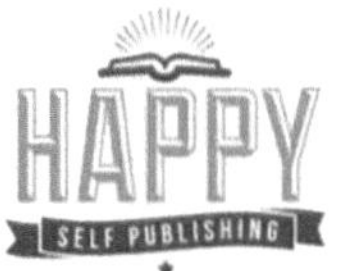

DISCLAIMER

The advice and strategies found within may not be suitable for every situation. This work is produced and sold with the understanding that neither the author nor the publisher is held responsible for the results accrued from the advice in this book.

Copyright © 2018 by Beachhouse Publications

Publishing Services by Happy Self Publishing
www.happyselfpublishing.com

Year: 2018

No portion of this book may be reproduced, stored in a retrieval system, or transmitted in any forms or by any means – electronic, mechanical, photocopying, recording, scanning or other – except for brief quotations in critical reviews or articles, without the prior written permission of the author.

ISBN-13:9781796305159
ISBN-10:

DEDICATION

This book is dedicated to the Captain of Team Jill, my best friend and husband, James. Without your unwavering love and support, I would have given up a long time ago.

To my family who are also very supportive of me during my bad days. I hope you will always help me save my steps by helping me with the garden every Mother's Day.

CONTENTS

ACKNOWLEDGEMENTS

This book could not have been possible without the help from so many people.

First, my book coach, R.E. Vance. You gave me the 'push' I needed to get this book done.

My editor, Spencer Borup, your help has been amazing, and I hope this is just the beginning.

My accountability partner, La Taunya. Even though we've never met, I think this is the beginning of a great friendship.

And finally, to the members of my Launch Team: Dad, Sam, Tracy, Karen, Wendy, Brenda, Drema, Joel, Jennifer W., Vicki, Dawn, Corinne, Qat, Sheila, Angie, Dawn, Noah, John, Maureen, Jackie, Johnny, Aimee, and Jen.

INTRODUCTION

Chronic pain—millions of Americans live in pain. It comes in many forms, shapes, sizes, and definitions. But what is it like to "live *with* pain"?

In this book I'm going to give you an in-depth look at what it's like to live with chronic pain. You'll see the good, the bad, and the ugly.

You see, I'm one of the millions who live in chronic physical pain.

I am a highly educated Nurse Practitioner and college professor. When I turned eighteen, I joined my local fire department and became a firefighter. Soon after, I became an Emergency Medical Technician (EMT), and a couple years after that I became a paramedic and then a Registered Nurse. During my nursing career I worked in a steel mill and many different critical care units, as well as owned my own billing company. After being a nurse for ten years, I went back to school and became a Nurse Practitioner (NP).

The bulk of my NP career has been spent working with patients with leukemia and lymphoma and patients who had undergone a bone marrow or stem cell transplant. I've spent a total of eleven years as part of the Ohio Disaster Medical Assistance Team (OH-DMAT) where I was deployed to several disasters.

Yet despite all those years of hard work, I've suddenly had to alter every aspect of my life because of chronic pain. I've had to give up the activities that I loved, alter my motivation, and change my career path.

I am not alone. According to the National Center for Health Statistics, it is estimated that 76.2 million people suffer from chronic pain.

Let's put this into perspective: according to the Center for Disease Control, there are 30.3 million people with diabetes[1]. According to the American Heart Association, there are 18.7 million people with coronary heart disease (heart attack and chest pain) and stroke. Finally, according to the American Cancer Society, there will be 1.8 million people diagnosed with cancer in 2018[2].

Chances are, you currently live with chronic pain—and if you don't, you certainly know someone who does. Whatever the case, in this

---

[1] Of that 30.3 million, 23.1 million are diagnosed and 7.2 million are undiagnosed; of that same 30.3 million, 5 percent are type 1 diabetics, the other 95 percent type 2.

[2] www.painmed.org/files/facts-and-figures-on-pain.pdf

book I'm going to give you a peak behind the curtain of what it's like to function, cry, and thrive as someone whose every minute is impacted by chronic pain. You've never read the real truth about what life is like for someone who lives in chronic pain.

You may think that someone living with chronic pain is simply lazy and trying to get out of work. Or that they are a drug-seeker who is just looking for their next high.

This is NOT true.

This book will show you the day-to-day and minute-by-minute impact of chronic pain. You will learn ways that you or someone you love can overcome these challenges.

I promise you that after reading this book you will gain a fuller understanding of what a person goes through each day when living with chronic pain. You will discover simple low-cost and no-cost ways that you can modify your surroundings to improve your quality of life, and if your loved one suffers from chronic pain, you will learn ways that you can help and support this person.

The time is now. Don't suffer in silence any longer. You are not alone. There are ways to survive, cry, and *thrive*—despite chronic pain. Take control of your life right now . . . make it productive . . . and enjoy the new life you've created.

CHAPTER 1

STEPPING INTO MY DAY

My day starts around 4:30 a.m. every day, seven days a week, including holidays.

You see, for someone in chronic pain, there are no days off.

Every day is a day with pain.

You must carefully plan each hour of each day of each week of each year. One planning misstep will lead to a lost day due to intractable pain or a hungover feeling from taking your medicine for breakthrough pain.

We're only given so many days on this earth . . . I refuse to lose any of them to chronic pain.

I get up extra early so I can take my medicine, warm up my joints, and gently stretch. By getting up this early and taking my morning medicine, I'm also giving time for my medicine to start working. This way I can start my work day by 8:30 a.m.

If it's a "good" day, subjectively speaking, I can make my own coffee. Breakfast is usually just a protein bar—I don't want to waste my energy making breakfast so grabbing a protein bar is an easy fix. The day has just begun; I have to piece out my energies a little bit at a time so they will last all day. In my mind, making myself breakfast is a waste of good energy and will leave me on the couch for the evening or in bed by 8:00 p.m.

If you and I were to meet for the first time and you asked, "Tell me a little about yourself,: the first thing I would tell you is that I'm a Nurse Practitioner. I have a doctorate degree, which is ironic because I hated high school and skipped more than I ever went; I graduated high school early for that very reason. I'd also tell you that I loved being an NP and taking care of my patients.

"Loved" in the past tense because I am now a college professor. It's difficult to manage a patient when your every thought is consumed by your own pain, how much it hurts to walk, to sit, to stand. So I left full-time patient care to become a college professor.

My patients became peripheral targets of

my chronic pain. My patients hated it when I left. They wanted to come with me. They asked why I was leaving and, of course, I didn't dare tell them the truth. I was the invincible healer. I couldn't let my patients know that I was in severe pain. They were my patients and I was their healthcare provider, not their friend.

So, you see, when I left patient care and changed my career path, my patients lost someone they trusted with their lives. I was a very good clinician. It came naturally to me and I loved it. But that was to be no more. Chronic pain owned me now and I was helpless against it.

Or so I thought.

I still wonder about my patients and how they are doing. I hope they know that I didn't abandon them, that I still think of them, and that I still, truly care about them. Chronic pain took me away from them. Tangential damage.

What does my twenty-four-hour day look like now? After waking up and taking my medicine, I purposefully move. I stretch my back, my neck, my shoulders. I meditate to clear my head of bad thoughts. I pray for help to make it through another day. I hope that this day might just be the day that everything turns around. Today will be the day when the pain will be over, and I'll be "normal" again. Perhaps I'll be able to walk my dog around the block *and* be able to fix dinner for my husband!

Maybe. The day is just starting. Who knows?

I have the luxury of being able to work from home when I need to. Some days, the task of climbing a staircase to get to my closet and bathroom to get myself ready to go to work is insurmountable. If and when I do arrive at work, my office isn't set up to be the most comfortable for me.

At home I have a nice comfortable chair with a nice support pillow for my lower back. I take stretch breaks every hour and I can keep myself in a routine. For my chronic pain management, a routine is essential. Any straying from the routine requires planning ahead so that I have enough energy to make it through the day.

I usually work in short blocks of time. I cluster activities to conserve my energy. I make a list of everything that I need to get accomplished that day and then I prioritize them. I place the most important tasks at the top of the list so that, if by chance I run out of energy before my list is complete, I'll have the most important tasks accomplished.

Working from home also allows me to start my day earlier, since I don't have to spend my morning getting ready for work or commuting. I can answer emails, take a little break, answer more emails, then work on my "to do" list.

I set reminders to stand and stretch routinely. If I don't, inertia will take over and I'll be so stiff it will take me about twenty-five minutes to stand up straight. I also have reminders to take my medication throughout the day—otherwise the pain will overcome me and it will take several hours to get it under control.

I take a lot of supplemental vitamins and herbs in the hopes that one of these will be the "magic pill" that makes everything normal again. I hope that one day the chronic pain will ease up or a better way to manage the pain without side effects will be discovered. Maybe this is all a bad dream and when I wake up and the enduring pain will be gone.

Unfortunately, this isn't a dream. The pain is here to stay, so you must learn to cope with it. Planning out each day is one way to come to terms with it. Sure, you can ask yourself, "What if today is the day I wake up and I never have a day filled with pain again?" But more practical questions are: What if today is the day when your routine quits working? What if the stretching doesn't help? The medicine quits working? Then what?

I try to explain to outsiders what my day looks like through the eyes of pain. I tell them that at the beginning of each day I start with so many "steps." For every action that I make, I use up part of my bucket of steps.

Most people begin each day with limitless possibilities and the energy to do whatever they want. They don't worry about the effects of their actions.

But when you have chronic pain, you start each day with a certain amount of energy—or "steps." For example, I start my day with ten steps in my bucket. Each task that I do during my day is going to cost me a step. Getting ready for work isn't as simple as just brushing my teeth, putting on mascara, and getting dressed. In my case, this means getting up early (hoping that I was able to get a slight reprieve from pain by enjoying a restful night's sleep), stretching, taking morning medicine, and grabbing a protein bar. These simple steps will cost me one "step."

Then I shower, shave my legs, towel off, dry my hair, and brush on some mascara (hoping to camouflage the dark circles under my eyes). This will cost me another step. This is a lot of movement for a morning and more often than not will actually cost me *two* steps—but for this analogy, we will only use one.

Next, I choose something to wear to work. Not as easy as it sounds! The level of pain I'm in that morning has a great impact on what I'll wear that day. What I can physically put on by myself that day must be taken into consideration. Pantyhose are completely unmanageable. Socks that come up past my ankles are always out—they aggravate the neuropathy in my legs. Shoes that tie or zip are also out—I can't reach down there to tie or zip them (I have a long-handled shoehorn that I use every day to get my slip-on shoes on). I also have to put a Lidoderm patch on my back (I've gotten really good at doing this by myself with the aid of the doorframe—imagine a bear scratching its back on a tree). Another patch goes on my right groin and a small, air-activated hand warmer goes on my right foot because the foot stays frozen all the time (I buy these things by the case because I go through two a day).

All of this takes two steps.

Now, two hours later I've used up four steps—and I haven't even left my house yet! Not to mention how depressed and frustrated I feel because it's taken me this long to get ready for work. I now make a choice about how to use the rest of my steps, because once my steps are gone, they're gone. If I borrow steps from tomorrow, I'll be left with less steps to work with tomorrow, and the next day, and the next, until my bucket of steps is completely empty.

I've done this many times; these are very bad days for me and my family. I'm not a nice person to be around during these times.

Heaven forbid I get sick. What if I catch a cold? That will use up more steps. Steps that I have already carefully allotted a specific use for each. What if I want to go to the movies tomorrow evening? I must save steps for that too. All events, good and bad, take extra steps that have been specifically designated for a daily task, such as going upstairs to take a shower.

I plan every day and every task. I write down every appointment and keep detailed records and notes. What if my mind is too busy trying to shut out the pain that I forget a meeting or an appointment? Thus, the detailed notes and calendar appointments.

I carry a book bag to work. It's better for me ergonomically and I can put more stuff in it. "Stuff" is usually a three-ring binder, packed lunch (more about that later), disposable air-activated hand warmers, packets of Biofreeze, Excedrin, pens, highlighters, a portable phone charger (also more about that later), a bottle of water, a notebook, and my daily planner. I still carry a handbag that has my identification in it along with the keys to the office, breath mints, earphones for my cellphone, more pens, mascara, eyeliner, a small notebook in case I need to write something down, a small pack of tissues, another air-activated hand warmer, my remote to turn on my spinal stimulator, and extra batteries for the remote.

I go to work about one day a week. It's about a twenty-minute drive, which goes by very quickly because I listen to audiobooks or inspirational podcasts. Once I arrive at work, I get to park close to the building because of my special parking permit. I used to be embarrassed about this, but now I realize that I save a tiny amount of energy by parking closer.

And energy is a resource more precious than gold.

My office is on the fourth floor. I never take the stairs—that could be suicidal if I trip and fall. And my office is close to the elevator—another small blessing. However, the elevator seems to be the only close-by amenity. I had to buy a small refrigerator and microwave for my office, as well as a printer. Walking back and forth down the hallway all day to warm up lunch or retrieve print jobs uses up three or four steps from my bucket—too many to waste!

There are several very good places to eat and get a great cup of coffee, but walking to those places is going to use up a step that has not been designated for that purpose on that day. So I pack my lunch, drink my coffee at home, and keep refillable water bottles in my small refrigerator so I always have something to drink (some of the medicine I take leaves me with a dry mouth).

I usually go to work for meetings which are held in different places around campus. These places always require walking—and, therefore, steps from my bucket—to get to. Most days I walk slow with a small stride because of the pain.

I don't take the stairs and get embarrassed when people ask, "You're okay to take the stairs—right?" I jokingly tell them, "No, I'm too old." People comply, but I know they are looking at me like, "Yeah . . . right. Lazy."

Going to each meeting will take at least one step, depending on proximity.

Two meetings? Two steps.

When my day is over, I pack up my book bag—it's usually heavier when I leave work than when I arrived for whatever reason. I go out to my car, load everything in, and take off for home.

I have had several physical therapists tell me to "pack less" because I'm "hurting my back."

No, you have it backward—I have to pack so much *because* I have a hurt back!

I've tried to take items out of my handbag

that I don't need, but taking out that extra pen didn't seem to make that much difference in weight to me. Everything in my bag is carefully chosen because I need it.

The tissues and mascara? To wipe up tears and to hide the redness in my eyes from crying.

The remote for the spinal stimulator? Keeps the edge off. I use it every day.

The extra batteries? I was caught with dead batteries in the stimulator's remote control once—and I'll never do *that* again.

The phone charger? I keep an extra phone-charging cord in my car . . . but if I don't have to walk out to the car to retrieve it, I've saved myself a step!

My total workday has used up four steps from the bucket. Add that to my two-step morning routine and I'm left with only four steps in my bucket to use to drive home, feed the dogs, feed the husband, change my clothes, wash my face, and unwind . . . if I have enough steps left.

This is a "normal" day. If the pain is worse than normal, the day is a crapshoot.

My days are never consistently "normal." The one constant is that I'm always mad at my lack of control and lack of productivity.

If I have a special event to attend that evening, I have to cut something out of my normal day so that I will have enough steps left for the special event. Special events include going to local fairs, craft shows, an after-work event, or even a farmer's market.

People with chronic pain usually experience a loss of the life they once knew. In my case, I have had to totally turn my life in a different direction.

Facts and Figures

What is chronic pain?

According to the American Academy of Pain Medicine (AAPM), chronic pain is *pain that persists.*

"Pain signals keep firing in the nervous system for weeks, months, even years. There may have been an initial mishap such as a sprained back, serious infection, or there may be an ongoing cause of pain such as arthritis, cancer, or an ear infection, but some people suffer chronic pain in the absence of any past injury or evidence of body damage. Many chronic pain conditions affect older adults. Common chronic pain complaints include headache, lower back pain, cancer pain, arthritis pain, neurogenic pain (pain resulting from damage to the peripheral nerves or to the central nervous system itself), and psychogenic pain (pain not due to past disease or injury or any visible sign of damage inside or outside the nervous system)."[3]

Twenty-five million adults endure chronic pain on a daily basis, and of these, 23 million report pain so intense they are unable to work or care for themselves.[4]

Evidence

People with chronic pain die at a 50 percent higher rate over ten years than those without pain.

Also, chronic pain is a significant financial burden. Individuals with chronic pain incur, on average, $10,000 per year in medical expenses, costing the U.S. at least $600 billion per year in healthcare and disability costs.[4]

Call to Action

If you suffer from chronic pain, here is something you can do to start your day off right:

Stretching is a no-cost way to get your joints loosened up. According to *Prevention*

---

[3] AAPM Facts and Figures on Pain
http://www.painmed.org/patientcenter/facts_on_pain.aspx
[4] Arnstein, P., St. Marie, B., & Zimmer, P.A. (2017). Nurse Practitioner Healthcare Foundation Managing Chronic Pain with Opioids: A Call for Change, 2017

magazine[5] there are five stretches you can do each morning, in less than five minutes, even before getting out of bed!

1. *Full-body stretch*: On an inhale, reach your arms overhead, clasp your fingers together, flip your palms out toward the wall behind your head, and push your palms away from you. At the same time, reach your toes away from your arms, keeping your knees straight. Hold this fully stretched position for five counts, then exhale and release the stretch. Repeat three times total.

2. *Figure-four stretch*: Cross your right foot over your left knee, making the shape of the number 4. Slowly bend your left knee up toward the ceiling, either keeping the left foot on your mattress or hugging it in toward your chest. Be sure to keep your right knee bent out to the right as you try to maintain this shape. Hold for five deep breaths, then switch sides.

3. *Knees-to-chest stretch*: From a supine position, bend your knees until the soles of your feet are on the bed. Use your hands to draw one knee in toward your chest at

---

[5] https://www.prevention.com/fitness/do-these-stretches-before-getting-out-of-bed/slide/1

a time, wrapping your arms around both shins. Relax your head on your pillow and hold this "self-hug" for ten deep breaths.

4. *Supine twist*: From the knees-to-chest stretch, release your grip of your shins and let your arms fall out to a T shape on either side of your torso. Use your core to guide your legs over to rest on one side, keeping your knees bent and shoulders planted down into your mattress. If it's easy on your neck, gaze toward the opposite side. Hold for ten deep breaths, then repeat on the other side.

5. *Seated forward bend*: Begin by lifting your torso upright from a reclined position. Keeping your legs straight, inhale and lengthen through your spine; as you exhale, start to walk your fingertips toward your feet. Keep lengthening your spine with your inhalation and sink a bit deeper into this seated forward fold with your exhalation. When you get to your farthest point, let your neck hang heavy toward your legs, releasing any tension. After ten rounds of breath, slowly lift your torso back up.

CHAPTER 2

AM I JUST GETTING OLD?

You reach a certain age in life and your body starts changing. Gravity takes effect and skin begins sagging, muscles don't look as toned as they once did, and you start to wake up stiff and achy for no reason.

Now imagine that you wake up several times in the middle of the night just to turn over because of pain. When morning finally does come, you're still just as tired as you were before you went to bed—and you realize you can't stand up straight because your back is so stiff. You try to put on your slippers but you can't reach your feet from the pain.

Maybe you're just getting older. That's what everyone tells you.

"Oh, you're just getting older. Wait until you reach *my* age! Then you'll really know what pain is like!"

Great.

You, however, know that this isn't simply *aging*.

You know that you want to go downstairs and make a cup of coffee, but managing the stairs when you're this stiff, sore, and achy is a major undertaking. What if you fall down the stairs? You'll end up with broken bones and spending days in the hospital.

For now, you sit on the edge of your bed, put on a pair of elastic-waist yoga pants, slip your toes into your shoes, and then hold on to the stair rail for dear life and slowly make your way down the stairs.

This is my morning routine every day. Whether I'm at home, at a conference for work, or on vacation. Every night I toss and turn because the pain robs me of my sleep and every morning is met with one question.

How am I going to get through this day?

What exactly is pain? According to the American Academy of Pain Medicine (AAPM), pain can be *acute* or *chronic*. Acute pain is a normal sensation triggered in the nervous system to alert you to possible injury.[6] Chronic pain can be the result of injury or disease, or the disease itself.

Chronic pain remains for days—or, more often, for years.

With chronic pain, the pain signals keep firing in the nervous system for weeks, months, or even years. The chronic pain may be the consequence of injury or body damage. Many people think that chronic pain goes hand-in-hand with aging. But chronic pain does not discriminate. Young and old alike can be a victim to chronic pain.

For some, chronic pain may be the result of an injury, such as a back strain, or even an infection. Sometimes chronic pain is the result of an ongoing condition, such as cancer or arthritis. However, some people suffer from chronic pain without any past injury or body damage.

The cause of my pain, for example, is from a rare condition called "adhesive arachnoiditis"—a progression of the inflammatory condition, arachnoiditis—and before you make a joke, it has nothing to do with spiders. Adhesive arachnoiditis is known as one of the worst pain

---

[6] AAPM Facts and Figures on Pain
http://www.painmed.org/patientcenter/facts_on_pain.aspx

conditions to have, along with metastatic bone cancer.[7]

The National Organization of Rare Disorders describes arachnoiditis as "a disease characterized by an acute inflammatory stage that occurs in the *dura* (exterior) and the *arachnoid* (interior), two of the three membranes that cover and protect the brain, the spinal cord, and the nerve roots. The arachnoid layer contains the cerebrospinal fluid, which circulates from the brain to the *sacral* (your tailbone) area about every two hours."

The arachnoid membrane acts as a filter. It keeps things from invading the brain and spinal cord. Sometimes scarring occurs on the arachnoid membrane, which causes the nerve roots to clump together. If your nerve roots are stuck together, they can't do their job properly.

There are many theories as to why a person gets adhesive arachnoiditis. Among the most popular ones are injuries to the area from repeat spinal operations and trauma to the spinal cord. I've never had back surgery or any other invasive procedure, yet I'm one of the rare people who have had adhesive arachnoiditis show up on several MRIs.

Adhesive arachnoiditis is incurable; it may

---

[7] https://practicalpainmanagement.com

progressively get worse, in fact, or it may not. For me, it has progressively gotten worse. What started with low back pain now includes right groin pain, a right foot that stays ice cold 100 percent of the time, and stabbing "hot-poker" sensations in my right thigh.

I keep a walker that converts into a wheelchair in the back of my car for bad days, or for when I want to go anywhere that may require a lot of walking or standing still for longer than two minutes.

Adhesive arachnoiditis is not directly fatal; however, there have been cases of suicide due to the despair of unrelieved pain.

According to the National Pain Report, one in every three Americans lives with pain. Pain has been called the "great equalizer" because it knows no gender, race, or religion.

Every day, those of us with pain fight. We fight to take a step, to get out of bed, and to live a normal life. In the end, we learn we must develop a new normal; a normal that includes pain in our day-to-day functions.

Pain, if left untreated, can have many side-effects. People with persistent pain can become irritable, short-tempered, and impatient. It's no wonder! The person suffering from unrelenting pain finds it difficult to focus on anything *but* their pain. Sounds frustrating, right?

Facts and Figures

Where is the most commonly reported site of pain? The low back, followed by migraine pain and then neck pain.

For Americans under the age of forty-five, low back pain is the leading cause of disability. Adults with low back pain are often in worse physical and mental health than people who do not have pain. These individuals are also more than four times as likely to experience serious psychological distress as people without low back pain.[8]

For many people with chronic pain, it is difficult to find solutions or workarounds to simple, everyday problems.[9] A traffic jam, which most people would be mildly annoyed by but ultimately take in stride, could seriously throw off the routine of someone who is putting forth so much effort just to get through the day.

After a while, these daily interruptions wear you down. Your energy is nonexistent and your motivation has been depleted.

People with chronic pain will limit their social interactions in an effort to reduce stress and to

---

[8] National Center for Health Statistics. Health, United States, 2016: *With Chartbook on Long-term Trends in Health*. Hyattsville, MD. 2017.
[9] http://www.ipcaz.org/long-term-effects-untreated-chronic-pain/

decrease the amount of energy they have to spend reacting to their environment. Because of this, many people with chronic pain develop symptoms that mimic depression or they develop true depression. Depressive symptoms include lack of interpersonal interaction, difficulty concentrating on simple tasks, the desire to simplify their life as much as possible, and isolation. They may start sleeping a lot because this makes the pain less intrusive.

Recent studies[10] have shown that chronic pain can actually affect a person's brain chemistry, their immune system, and even change the wiring of the nervous system. Cells in the spinal cord and brain of a person with chronic pain, especially in the section of the brain that processes emotion, weaken quicker than normal. This can aggravate the depression-like symptoms.

Because of this, it's easy to see why it becomes harder for people with chronic pain to process multiple issues at once and react to ongoing changes in their environment. Sleep is more difficult because the section of the brain

---

[10] McGill University. (2016, January 28). Chronic pain changes our immune systems: Epigenetics may bring us a step closer to better treatments for chronic pain. *ScienceDaily*. Retrieved from
www.sciencedaily.com/releases/2016/01/160128074319.htm

that regulates the sleep cycle is impacted by chronic pain. The sleep regulator becomes smaller from reacting to the pain, making falling asleep more difficult for people with chronic pain[11].

This change in a person's brain chemistry can cause the person to experience anxiety. After repeated episodes of recurring pain, the brain rewires itself to anticipate future bouts, which makes patients constantly on the lookout for worsening pain, which in turn can lead to anxiety.

All of these side effects can make the chronic pain sufferer feel hopeless. In fact, about one-third of patients with chronic pain will feel despair at some point during their lifetime.

Call to Action

I know all the information above sounds bleak. So what can you do to help?

Writing, scribing, or journaling may help you or someone you know with chronic pain to keep track of your pain level and possible "triggers." According to Dictionary.com, a *trigger* is something that will cause a situation or event to

---

[11] http://www.ipcaz.org/long-term-effects-untreated-chronic-pain/

happen. For some people, a trigger might be a change in the weather, such as a rainy or cool day. Or it may be moving a certain way or doing a specific exercise.

Every morning, write down your level of pain. One of the most common ways to do this is with a simple pain scale. The scale starts at 0 and ends at 10, with 0 being no pain and 10 being the worst pain you've ever had in your life. Many pain clinics will use this same scale; each time you go to your appointment, you will be asked to "rate" your pain for that day. By writing down your level of pain on a daily basis, you may start to notice trends in how you feel related to certain events.

When your pain is rated higher than normal, reflect on the previous forty-eight hours of activity and/or weather-related events.

Did you lift something heavy?

Try a new exercise?

Move in a way that is not common for you?

Was yesterday a "good pain day," and perhaps you did a little too much?

You should also take a look at the weather. Yes, the weather! If your joint pain is worse when it's cold or raining, it's not your imagination. You may be less active in cooler weather. Decreased activity can lead to increased stiff joints and pain.

On top of that, however, changes in barometric pressure can cause some people to have worsening pain, possibly because the change in barometric pressure affects joint pressure[12]. As the temperature increases and a high-pressure system moves in, this will increase the barometric pressure and ease the pain.

A study by Timmermans et al. (2015)[13] found that humidity may also impact pain. The study included more than 800 adults living in one of six European countries, each adult having osteoarthritis of the hip, knee, or hands. Even though changes in weather did not seem to affect symptoms, higher humidity was linked with increasing pain and stiffness, especially in colder weather.

Start writing down your daily pain level, check the weather, and write down any other unusual or new activity that you may have done to trigger a flare in your pain. Over time you will start to notice trends in your pain level and changes in the weather, or if the new activity

---

[12] https://www.prevention.com/health/pain-management-common-myths-debunked

[13] Timmermans, E.J., Schaap, L.A., Herbolsheimer, F., Dennison, E.M., Maggi, S., Pedersen, N.L.,...EPOSA Research Group. (2015). The influence of weather conditions on joint pain in older people with osteoarthritis: Results from the European Project on OSteoArthritis. *Journal of Rheumatology, 42,* 1885-92. Doi: 10.3899/jrheum.141594

you've incorporated into your life has made a difference in your pain level. You may be able to notice positive trends as well. Maybe your new relaxation technic has helped you to be more active?

Or maybe the morning stretches help you feel motivated and energized all day long!

CHAPTER 3

NO, IT'S NOT A FEAR OF SPIDERS

When I wake up each morning, I stretch before getting out of bed. I start with my feet and work my way up. I rotate my ankles, bend and straighten my legs, arch and straighten my back, shrug my shoulders, and stretch my arms overhead. This routine takes about ten minutes.

Then, it takes me about twenty minutes every morning to stand up straight.

I put on my socks and slippers and slowly make my way downstairs. It could be ninety-five degrees outside and I have to put on socks and slippers. To an outsider, I'm positive that this routine looks comical. To me, it's just a normal part of my day.

Going downstairs also takes longer than normal. I go down one stair at a time, hoping that I don't miss a step and that my slippers stay firmly on so I don't trip and fall.

I methodically count the stairs so I know when I'm getting close to the bottom. My back is still too stiff at this point to be able to look down at the stairs—so I count them. Thirteen. Thirteen lucky stairs from top to bottom. (Thankfully, I'm not superstitious or I would have to move!)

The stairs are carpeted and we have a handrail—thank goodness! I heavily rely on both. My parents used to live in a house with uncarpeted, wooden stairs that my mother kept highly polished, and that had no railing. Those stairs are very intimidating to someone who isn't steady on their feet!

I've never fallen down the stairs in my house, but I do experience at least one nasty fall a year. Last year's fall was in an auditorium that was packed full of people. I was at an event that was just finishing up and I fell down the stairs and landed on a large metal pole, everything in my purse tumbled out. I ended up with a large, painful bruise from my left collar bone all the way down to my left ankle. A trip to the emergency room, some X-rays, an EKG, and CT scans showed nothing broken, but there was a lot of swelling and a lot of embarrassment.

Once I reach the main floor of my house, I head into the kitchen and, turning on my spinal stimulator, I take my morning concoction of medications and supplements so they can start working their way through my body and help me loosen up.

I saunter over to the coffee machine and make my first cup of coffee for the day. Some mornings are worse than others, and some are better. Either way, I have to get up two hours earlier than needed so that I can loosen up and medications can take effect.

As I said in Chapter 1, I purchase air-activated hand warmers by the case. Because of the nerve damage in my back, I have "sensory neuropathy." This means that the affected area—in this case, my foot—stays ice cold all the time.

It can be 100 degrees outside and my foot will still be freezing. I don't have the "pins-and-needles" sensation that is typical of neuropathy; instead, I have to keep an air-activated hand warmer on top of my foot twenty-four hours a day, seven days a week. I used to love to wear sandals and flip-flops, but I can't anymore—instead, I have to wear socks and put the warmers on top of the socks. I wear the warmers to bed and sometimes wear two socks on each foot just to keep warm.

I used to put the warmer directly on my foot, but then I burnt my foot and had a terrible blister for almost a month. At the time, I didn't even feel the warmer burning my skin. Lately, the neuropathy has gotten worse and it feels like I'm constantly stepping in something wet. I have four dogs, so at first I thought I was stepping in dog urine. That wasn't the case. Just another exciting symptom to deal with.

Fortunately, I do have good blood flow to the foot, unlike many neuropathy patients—but my right foot still stays ice cold. The only times I don't have warmers on my feet is when I'm at swim class or in the shower. This also means that I have to keep an extra warmer with me everywhere I go—but more on that later.

Adhesive arachnoiditis (AA) is what is called an "invisible illness." To a stranger I look "normal." I don't have the contorted joint deformity of someone with severe arthritis, or the stiffened extremities of someone with a joint replacement. I don't have the tell-tale scar down the center of my knee that screams, "I have an artificial knee joint!"

And I'm not alone. Many people suffer from chronic pain that is invisible.

Facts and Figures

According to the American Academy of Pain Medicine,[14] pain affects more Americans than heart disease, diabetes, and cancer combined. It is estimated that 100 million Americans suffer from chronic pain.

Even if you're not one of the 100 million sufferers, the burden of chronic pain still impacts you. The emotional and physical costs of caring for a loved one in pain and the financial cost due to disability, lost wages, and productivity is estimated to be between $560 and $635 billion. Approximately 42 million Americans report that pain disrupts their sleep a few nights a week, and 50 to 75 percent of patients die in moderate to severe pain.

Call to Action

There are several modifications you can make to counteract some of the physical discomforts associated with pain. Using air-activated hand warmers are one way that I manage my chronically cold foot, as well as a heating pad within easy reach for my back or other achy joints.

---

[14] http://www.painmed.org/patientcenter/facts_on_pain.aspx

If heat doesn't work for you, you can try cold therapy. I keep reusable icepacks in my freezer to use on other achy areas. I simply put a washcloth on the area where I'm going to put the icepack, and then lay the icepack on top of the washcloth. It's important to remember not to put the icepack directly on your skin so that you don't damage or injure your skin. (Remember my blistered toe?)

Since bending over is difficult—if not impossible—for me, I keep a long-handled shoehorn hanging by the front door to help me slip on my shoes. Most of my shoes are slip-ons, but on the rare occasion when I can wear a pair with shoestrings, I double-knot them so I won't trip on untied laces and then have to figure out how to retie them—I might not be able to bend over and reach them later.

Another indispensable aide is a "grabber." A grabber is a tool with a long handle and rubberized jaws that will allow you to simply squeeze the handle to activate the jaws and pick something up. Mine even has magnets at the tips of the jaws so that I can pick up small metal objects, such as a straight pin. I keep this within easy reach so that I can easily pick up items and not trip over them.

CHAPTER 4

I'M EXHAUSTED FROM TRYING TO FEEL BETTER

The other day I told my husband that I don't like going to sleep each night because I'm never sure what the next day will bring. I may wake up in the morning feeling great and I think, "Finally! This is it! The day that I've been waiting for! The pain is tolerable! Life is going to be nothing but rainbows and unicorns!" Or I might wake up the next day and the pain is much worse. "Finally! This is it! The day that I've been dreading—I can't make it down my thirteen stairs."

I go to bed every night hoping that the morning will bring something new. Maybe I've just been having a nightmare all this time and when I wake up, I'll be able to do the things that I used to do. Just maybe.

I go to bed night after night with this thought in my mind. Then, morning after morning I wake up, bent over and stiff-jointed. Because of this, I dread the night. I know that getting a good night's sleep is a toss-up.

Maybe I'll be able to rest, but more likely I won't. I wake up when I need to change positions because turning from side to side isn't a simple task. I have to hold on to something to help me turn because it hurts too much. And, more often than not, when I wake up, the pain will still be there—it's not a nightmare, it's reality. I can't judge how bad my day is going to be until I try to stand up. Then, my morning routine begins.

There are some nights when I'm awake more than asleep. It's impossible to find a position of comfort no matter how hard I try. I've tried different mattresses, mattress covers, sleeping on something hard, sleeping on something soft, sleeping in a recliner, sleeping on the couch. It's a crap shoot. There's no rhyme or reason. If I don't get adequate rest, I take a short nap to give me the stamina to make it through the day.

Every evening, not knowing if I'm going to be able to sleep and how I'm going to wake up causes a lot of emotional turmoil. I get mad about what I can't control and I am apprehensive about the unknown. The anger will last for days. It sucks me into its grip and holds on for dear life. I get angry at the pain, angry because I can't do what I want to do, and angry because other people are allowed to live a normal life but I can't.

The anger spills into my personal relationships too. I often wonder how my family puts up with me during those times. I consider myself lucky because they tolerate my bad moods. I haven't found a cure for the anger. I know that as time passes, the anger will ebb until the next flare-up.

There are a lot of other emotions that go along with being in chronic pain. Some people may feel worthless because of pain. Or they may feel like they aren't a contributing member of society any more.

Or they may feel like they can't contribute to their family any more. Their pain may have taken away their livelihood or their sense of "being." The mere act of "being" has become too emotionally painful for them.

Often people who suffer from chronic pain "don't look sick." We look "normal" because there isn't an obvious outward deformity. I've had people tell me over and over again how "well you hid your pain." I think many people with chronic pain don't hide it—we just deal with it because the alternative is not dealing with it and who knows what that will do to us.

People don't see me crying so often that suicidal thoughts go through my head. They don't see my stash of urinary incontinent pads in my purse because there are many days where I'm incontinent. They don't see me struggling just to stand up because my groin is throbbing. They don't know that every four weeks I go to the doctor, every other week I see my counselor, and that every day is a complicated dance of pills, creams, patches, and heating pads. Only I see all of that.

I have a disability parking placard that I use because it's difficult for me to walk long distances. I've had my "special parking pass" for several years. I remember when I first got it and put it in my car. I remember being ashamed because I "didn't look sick."

What was I going to say when someone asked me why I had the disability parking sticker? What was I going to say when someone said, "You don't look sick" or "You don't look like you need that."

One day I was talking to some friends and the subject of the disability parking pass came up. My friends didn't realize that I used one. They proceeded to say how "so many people took advantage of the blue parking pass and they're not even handicapped! They're usually just fat!"

I was astonished! Would my friends say this if they knew the truth? Would they be saying this in front of me if they knew that I had one of those blue parking passes?

I'm not a person who shies away from controversy or difficult subjects. So, I told my friends: "I have one." At first, they didn't know what I was referring to, so I told them: "A disability parking permit."

At this point there was no turning back, so I told them that I have a progressive spinal condition and that walking long distances is very difficult for me. I also told them that I keep a walker and wheelchair in my car because when my husband and I go to festivals, I can't walk long enough to enjoy them—so, out comes the wheelchair!

Stunned silence followed by the obligatory apology, "We're so sorry. We had no idea. You've done a really good job of hiding it."

I considered it a teaching moment. I'm sure they considered it a learning moment for a whole different reason: "Treat Jill extra nice because she has a 'condition.' "

Perfect—now everyone is feeling the right amount of uncomfortableness. Score two for Team Jill! I'd rather be able to just use my wheelchair when I need it and not feel like I have to constantly justify myself to my friends—or strangers.

Don't get me wrong, there are benefits to using a wheelchair: I don't have to stand in lines at the airport—I'll tell you about the "incident" at Baltimore's airport later. And, I got a pass from the National Park Service to get into all the National Parks for free.

Score three for Team Jill!

Team Jill is a concept that was created by my husband when I first started to realize that I was going to be in pain for the rest of my life. It is his way of letting me know that he is always supportive of me.

I learned about Elisabeth Kübler-Ross's[15] stages of grief while I was in nursing school. The first stage is shock and denial.

My diagnosis wasn't all of a sudden. It was a gradual escalation of ongoing pain and other vague symptoms. It took months of doctor visits, X-rays, and procedures to try and figure out why my back hurt so much all of the time. Without a working diagnosis, the doctors weren't sure how to fix it.

I continued to expect that I would eventually

---

[15] Kübler-Ross, E. (1969). Five stages of grief: Kubler-ross model for death and bereavement counselling, personal change and trauma.

wake up pain-free. Denial can be an efficient way to cope in change in the beginning, but staying too long in this phase can be hazardous to your mental health. Shock can provide protection emotionally by reducing the feeling of being overwhelmed. The first stage can last for weeks.

The second stage of grieving is pain and guilt.[15] For someone who is grieving the loss of their previous health status, emotional pain and unnecessary guilt are the basis of stage two. Emotional pain, according to clinical psychologist Edwin Schneidman,[16] is "how much you hurt as a human being. It is mental suffering; mental torment."

Do you ever have conversations with yourself in your head? Do you ask yourself, "What have I done to deserve this? Why do I have to suffer from pain? Why can't my life just be normal?" Those conversations are a form of mental torment.

You might even think that God is "paying you back" for something that you've done or haven't done in your life. You might think, "If only I'd exercised more . . . or been nicer in fifth grade." You get the idea. You feel unnecessary

---

16 Shneidman ES. *The Suicidal Mind*. Oxford University Press; 1996. Appendix A Psychological Pain Survey. p. 173.

guilt for any number of reasons that, in the long run, have nothing to do with the chronic pain you're feeling today.

The third stage of grief is anger and bargaining.[15] The guilt you've been feeling gives way to anger. You get mad because you hurt. You get mad because the pain interrupts your plans and your life. You get mad because you're stuck waiting in the doctor's office for hours.

You yell at friends, your husband, your kids, your pets, and everyone else for no reason at all. The anger can become all-consuming. Relationships may suffer temporarily or even permanently. Bottled up emotions explode.

It's normal to ask, "Why me?" during this phase. You might even try bargaining—I know I have. "If I can only have one good day, I promise that I won't complain about the five bad days."

The fourth stage of grieving is depression, reflection, and loneliness.[15] During this phase, you find yourself looking back on what once was. During this stage, I remembered being able to go hiking (which I love), going on a long bicycle ride, and being able to stand longer than five minutes without pain.

When I start listing all of the activities that I can no longer participate in, I become depressed. I don't want to get dressed. I don't want to leave the house. I just want to curl up on the sofa and do nothing.

When I see my friends training for a ten-mile charity bicycle ride or planning a horseback riding trip, I feel isolated and lonely. I want to be able to ride in the charity event and go horseback riding, but I can't because of the pain.

Well-meaning friends and family will say, "Just pull yourself up by your bootstraps."

Worst advice ever.

The chronic pain sufferer isn't able to just snap out of it. The chronic pain sufferer has to be flexible enough with their plans so that if the day starts to go downhill fast they can still survive. People who don't have chronic pain can't understand this. This can lead to isolation and depression.

Reflection, or looking back on the past, can be beneficial for the chronic pain sufferer. This can help you prepare for the future and help you accept the enormity of your loss.

Working through these feelings, whether this is done by journaling, counseling, or meditating, can help you plan for the future and your new normal.

The fifth stage is known as the upward turn.[15] As you work through the sadness, depression, and isolation, you will "turn the corner," so to speak. You learn that there is a bit of blue sky among the gray; a light at the end of the tunnel; and that you can survive this by adapting.

The sixth stage is the reconstructive phase.[17] During this phase, your mind starts to accept the new you. You are able to identify rational solutions to daily issues such as putting on your socks and washing your hair. Tasks that seemed impossible become easier to manage.

You may learn that clustering your activities to save energy is a very workable strategy. Or you may realize that putting an empty, plastic trash bag on your car seat will help you slide in and out. These seemingly small victories will help you work through rebuilding and recreating your life and yourself.

The final stage is acceptance and hope.[17] Once you have learned to acknowledge and accept your new normal, you can move on.

Reaching this stage doesn't mean that everything is rosy, but it does allow you to feel hopeful for the future. You cannot go back in time, but you can reflect upon your past and move forward.

Acknowledgment of your situation will lead to planning. You will be able to plan to

---

[17] https://www.recover-from-grief.com

experience life again.

For me, this means that I can take a short stroll with my family, or that I can partake in one of my hobbies, such as painting furniture. My tasks may take longer to accomplish, but I've learned to accept this. It may take you months or years to get to this stage. But don't give up hope. You can and will work through this!

It takes a village. I need all the help I can get and I'm not afraid to ask for it. I need the help of my family members, coworkers, friends, professional counselors and physicians.

Remember the Baltimore Airport incident I mentioned earlier? My husband and I were standing in the TSA line at the Baltimore Airport. A few years ago, we were coming home from a combined business trip and mini-vacation.

My husband was with me—thank goodness or I probably would have ended up in jail! The TSA security line was very, very long and was moving at a snail's pace. This incident was before I was using a wheelchair to travel through the airport.

There was one TSA agent checking identification and there were probably seventy-five people in line to go through security. There was also another line for airport employees.

Person after person would go to the airport employee line and breeze right through without their identification or ticket being checked. Meanwhile, the line that my husband and I were in wasn't moving. After standing in line for an hour, I hit my breaking point.

My back was screaming in pain! I couldn't even stand up straight. There wasn't any place to sit except on the floor—but then it would be a major undertaking to help me up.

I yelled to the sole TSA agent and said, "Hey! I've been standing here for an hour and this line isn't moving. You're letting everyone go through the airport employee line without even checking! Can you get someone else to check identification?!"

The TSA agent politely replied, "Ma'am, you have not been standing in the line for an hour."

I told him, "Yes, I have!"

Then, something amazing happened: the other people in line supported me.

They also started yelling to the TSA agent, telling him that they had been standing line for an hour and that there needed to be a second agent. Several people said they were afraid of missing their flights because of this.

About five minutes later, a second TSA agent came to help.

My husband jokingly whispered in my ear, "You're going to get strip-searched."

I replied (in my outdoor voice), "Fine! Let

them search me! I'll get naked right here!"

I heard another traveler yell out, "Yeah! I'll get naked too!" I'm pretty sure it wasn't just a sign of solidarity.

Naturally, when it was my time to go through security, I was given a full pat-down instead of just being able to walk through the body scanner. But I didn't mind. I was just glad they didn't arrest me. And every time since then, I have requested a wheelchair to get through the airport. I always offer to show them my Medtronic card that has my stimulator information on it, because I "don't look sick" and sometimes I can actually feel the stares of other passengers as I sit in my wheelchair.

It was nice to be supported by a group of strangers. Even more important, it is nice to be supported by my family. As I mentioned before, my husband came up with the concept of Team Jill.

My family and close friends are all part of Team Jill. If I'm having a bad pain day and feeling desperate, tearful, and even suicidal, I can call or text one of my team members and talk, cry, or just lean on them.

The Team Jill concept is a way to remember to keep priorities where they need to be and to remind me that I don't need to sweat the small stuff. We assess situations as a team and decide how our decisions will impact my future with pain together. For example, we currently live in a two-story house, but when we get older, we will buy a ranch so that I won't have to navigate stairs. We buy cars that sit up higher so that it's easier to get in and out of them. Even something as simple as meal preparation is part of Team Jill. When I'm having a "good" pain day, members of my team will help me make freezer meals. These are meals or ingredients that we prepare ahead of time in order to make meal time easier. We usually make ten to fifteen freezer meals at a time. This makes future meal preparation so much easier.

Create *your* team of supporters. Keep those people close and be honest with them. Tell them when you're sad, frustrated, or angry. Let them know when you're just tired of being tired. Tell them the truth.

They can't help you if they don't know the full story, so keep them in-the-know.

CHAPTER 5

GETTING RID OF MY STILETTOS

I cry at all weddings. Tears of happiness and tears of joy. Looking at a bride and groom and all their happiness just makes me cry.

My oldest son got married a few years ago to a wonderful woman. I was so proud to be his mother and very proud of the young man he had become. I wore a nice, comfortable outfit at the wedding and decided to wear shoes that had a small heel.

The heel was only an inch—surely this wouldn't be a problem. Well, I was very wrong. That one-inch heel put me in so much pain that I had to leave the wedding early.

It wasn't because I was standing, it was because I did a lot of walking around in heels. I

53

don't normally wear heels so when I did, my back let me know that this was not acceptable.

My son quickly spoke to the disc jockey and rearranged the order of music so that we could do the mother-of-the-groom dance earlier and then I could leave. The following day was spent on the sofa. I never knew that something so small could cause so much pain. That was the last time that I've worn anything with a heel and I don't ever see that changing.

Having chronic back pain means that you need to change everything in your life. From the clothes and shoes you wear, to what kind of car you drive, and even what type of job you choose. The pain dominates all decisions.

Did you know that having chronic pain (and especially low back pain) determines what kind of car you drive? It's true. I drive an SUV, and I have for years. I am a car enthusiast and I used to drive cute little sports cars, but now I drive something that sits up a little higher—this makes it easier to get in and out. At this stage in my life, I think I could collapse myself into a cute little sports car, but I have no idea how I would get out of the car other than rolling out, so I'd have to live in the car—and that option isn't conducive to my current lifestyle.

Chronic pain also dictates what kind of shoes you wear. A few years ago, after a fall, one of my doctors told me to start wearing "sensible shoes." I'm not sure what he was referring to, because it's not like I wear four-inch stilettos. I conjured up an image of clunky shoes with Velcro straps.

I own only one pair of shoes that actually tie. They are a generic brand of exercise shoe and I wear them when I walk the dog. All of my other shoes are close-toed slip-ons.

There are other issues with shoes—I have a bad fall about once a year. I don't know if this is from neuropathy or clumsiness, but I take a nasty fall about once a year.

Another issue with shoes that don't slip on is actually getting your foot into the shoe so that you can lace, buckle, or zip the shoe. It takes me long enough to put on my socks, I can only imagine all the time I would lose by having to manipulate shoes every day. So, I'm resigned myself to wearing flat, slip-on shoes.

Having chronic pain doesn't just impact your choice of shoe or your choice of car. There are additional changes you must make when you have chronic pain. If you have arthritis in your hands, you have to wear clothes that are easy to put on and take off. You think about the size of the buttons and the ease of the zipper.

Careful consideration must also be given to the type of accessories you wear. Can you latch a necklace? Are your fingers going to swell around the ring? If you need to go the restroom in a hurry, will you be able to manipulate a buckle?

The type and location of your pain will depend on the modifications that you have to make. Thankfully, there are aids that you can purchase to help you with getting dressed or latching a bracelet.

People with chronic pain must also come to terms with the uncertainty of their symptoms. The day may start off pretty good and then, for whatever reason, you end the day in horrible pain. What do you do if you have a social engagement planned for that evening? You cancel. Many times, you have to cancel at the last minute. This makes it difficult for you and others to plan things.

My family and close friends understand this. However, there are times when I'm expected at an event in the evening and I absolutely cannot cancel at the last minute. So what do I do? I plan.

Planning for evening events begins one to two days before the actual event. Planning involves starting your day later than normal, so you have enough energy—or steps—to last until the evening. Or, you can delay other activities that you have planned so you'll be prepared for the evening. The freezer meals come in handy on these days.

It's imperative that you take care of yourself so you can fully participate in activities that occur later in the day. Leading up to the event, be sure that you're eating real, unprocessed foods, getting enough rest, and avoiding stressors that can strain the body. I've discovered that by taking care of myself and planning, that I can make it through evening activities.

Don't get me wrong, this doesn't ensure the boundless energy of a two-year-old, but it does help. Last summer when my husband and I went to Spain, I made sure that I ate freshly prepared food, avoided alcohol, and got a good night's rest so we could sight-see during the day.

By 5 p.m., I was ready to go back to our hotel; my husband would continue exploring the sights while I showered and rested and then he would bring back a delicious dinner. His support and understanding, and my careful planning gave us both a very enjoyable vacation.

Additional studies on people who have been diagnosed with osteoarthritis show that the physical and emotional complications of chronic pain also impact social activities. Also, patients with neuropathic pain have shown a decrease in physical functioning. This leads to irritability, negative emotions, and "feelings of anger which can have a negative impact on interpersonal relationships and levels of stress in families."[18]

Speaking from personal experience, I know that my neuropathy impacts my life every day. I don't have the kind of neuropathy that is common in someone who has diabetes—that pins and needles sensation. I have sensory neuropathy. Neuropathy is a disease of, or damage to the nerves. Sensory neuropathy is when you have damage to the nerves that provide feeling.

One night, several years ago, my husband and I were at a restaurant and suddenly, it felt like someone had stuck a hot poker in my mid-thigh on my right side. It was intense! I took in a very large gasp of air and everyone in the restaurant became dead silent.

My husband jumped up, convinced everyone that I was okay, and everyone went back to eating. I told my husband what I had just experienced, and we chalked it up to the way I was sitting coupled with the nerve problems from adhesive arachnoiditis.

---

[18] Dueñas, M., Ojeda, B., Salazar, A., Mico, J. A., & Failde, I. (2016). A review of chronic pain impact on patients, their social environment and the health care system. *Journal of Pain Research, 9*, 457–467. http://doi.org/10.2147/JPR.S105892

A few months later when we were taking our dogs for a walk around the block, that same hot-poker feeling happened again. The searing pain was so intense that I almost dropped to my knees. Once again, we attributed this to my adhesive arachnoiditis.

The frequency of the hot-poker sensation increased but now I also had a hard lump in the area where I was having these sudden jolts of pain. Now I was worried. I was working as a Nurse Practitioner in an oncology clinic that saw patients who had leukemia and lymphoma.

What if this hard knot that was causing this pain was the beginning of lymphoma? I'd seen stranger presenting symptoms for lymphoma, so I was concerned that this was cancer.

I called my family physician and made an appointment to be seen. He ordered some lab work and an x-ray of my right thigh and hip to see if there was something wrong internally. Everything came back normal. While this was good news, this was also frustrating; when you know that something is wrong and conventional medicine can't find it, it is very exasperating for the patient.

The hot-poker sensation continued without an official diagnosis, and was chalked-up to being an anomaly. But then, several months after the thigh pain began, I noticed that my right foot began to feel very cold. I could be wearing three pairs of socks and my right foot would still feel cold.

As a nurse who has spent several years working in intensive care units, I wanted to find the cause of these strange symptoms. The first thing that crossed my mind was a blood clot. But a blood clot didn't make a lot of sense because my foot didn't look like it wasn't getting blood flow.

I was perplexed and confused. What was going on with my body? Why was I having these painful and uncomfortable sensations?

I sent my pain physician an email telling him about my newest symptom and how this was concerning to me. I tried various ways of keeping my foot warm (wearing extra socks, putting the heating pad on it, etc.) but nothing lasted long-term.

Every time I go out in public, I'm afraid that I'm going to have that "hot poker" sensation again. I'm afraid that if it occurs again, I will yell so loud that I'll scare someone into having a heart attack. What if this happens when I'm in a movie? What if it happens when I'm attending a conference? Or giving a presentation? I'll draw a lot of very unwanted attention.

The next time I saw my pain physician, we reviewed my symptoms and he performed an exam of my foot. An ideal evaluation would be to get an MRI of the nerves and other structures in my back to see if my adhesive arachnoiditis was getting worse. But, because of the type of spinal stimulator that I have, I cannot have an MRI. I was given the diagnosis of sensory neuropathy.

Not knowing what is really causing these symptoms is very exasperating. If you have a diagnosis, you can work with that to make it better. But by not having a diagnosis, my physician is just making shots in the dark. This means that a lot of time is wasted by trying therapies that may or may not work.

I also worry that I'll get skin cancer on my foot because I keep this chemical warmer pressed against it 24/7. I also learned that I have no feeling on my second toe. One morning when I was getting ready for work, I noticed a large, fluid-filled blister on that toe. I had no idea that I had a blister there because I couldn't feel anything.

In 2016 Dueñas, Ojeda, Salazar, Mico, and Failde reviewed fifty-eight research studies that scientifically reviewed the impact of chronic pain on quality of life, activities of daily living, and family relationships. The results highlighted in the paper were many, but they were not surprising to those of us who suffer from chronic pain.

Dueñas et al. (2016) found that chronic pain emphatically impacted physical performance. In fact, they discovered that the ability to do intense physical activity, walk, carry out domestic chores, participate in social activities and maintain an independent lifestyle were the activities that were most affected.

There are also mental health repercussions, work-related consequences, diminished participation in social activities, and a strain on the entire health care system.

Chronic pain can have a lasting impact on one's social circle. Scientists are studying how biological factors such as genetics, psychological factors such as personality, and social factors such as culture, influence how we perceive chronic pain.

Chronic pain also impacts your sleeping patterns, fear, anxiety, depression, and coping mechanisms. All of these influence health-related quality of life and mental health.

When was the last time you got a good night's sleep? Did you toss and turn trying to find a position of comfort? Or were you woken up in the middle of the night because of your pain?

You're not alone. When you have chronic pain, it's very difficult to get the appropriate amount of good, high-quality sleep. When you haven't slept well, it's difficult to process other emotions such as fear, anxiety, and depression. It's difficult, if not impossible, to process emotions in a healthy manner. Studies[19] have shown that if you don't get enough sleep—thus becoming sleep deprived—you are more sensitive to pain. What's more, if you're anxious or depressed, it is harder to fall asleep and *stay* asleep.

Some chronic pain sufferers think that using alcohol to help sleep is the answer. It's not. Alcohol might temporarily numb the pain, but it interferes with normal sleep patterns and will end up making you even more sleep deprived, and you wake up even more cranky—not to mention the stress on your liver.

There are many ways to improve the quality of your sleep when you have chronic pain. One way is to reduce your level of stress. Don't be afraid to ask for help or to say "no" to people. You don't have to be all things to all people. Trust me. Someone else can run the bake sale, coach the softball team, or be the teacher's aide. You can even "outsource" your household chores. For example, where I live, I can order my groceries online and then drive to the store and

---

[19] Kundermann B., Krieg J.C., Schreiber W., & Lautenbacher S. (2004). The effect of sleep deprivation on pain. *Pain Research & Management, (9),* 25-32.

pick them up. I don't even have to get out of my car! They load the groceries for me. This saves me a lot of time and doesn't use up any steps from my bucket.

Another way to improve the quality of your sleep is to avoid caffeine before bedtime. You may even want to eliminate caffeine all together.

You can also try some mindfulness exercises; stretching before bed can help you relax. This can be done by focusing on deep breathing as you lie in bed. Some slow, deep breaths, in through your nose and out through your mouth, can help your body realize that it's time to slow down and rest.

When your sleep improves, your levels of anxiety and depression will also improve. Over time, this will lead to increased feelings of satisfaction and happiness.

In addition to proper sleep, it's important to fuel your body with the proper nutrients. Eating real food that doesn't contain chemical additives can help your body function at its maximum capacity.

Many people think that healthy food costs more. This isn't true. Unprocessed foods are more nutritious than processed foods. What are unprocessed foods? Think of anything that doesn't come in a box.

For protein, ground beef, chicken, tuna, cottage cheese, and eggs are all affordable sources. Frozen chicken breasts, tuna in cans, and cottage cheese are easy on the budget and provide the protein your body needs.

Carbohydrate choices include fresh fruits such as apples, bananas, and pears. You can also eat pasta and rice—just don't go overboard! Portion-control will help keep excess weight off. Frozen fruits and frozen vegetables are already prewashed, so this will save you time and energy.

Healthy fats are also an important part of a balanced diet. Examples of these include real butter, mixed nuts, and olive oil. You can also save money by buying the store brands.

Getting enough sleep and eating healthy will provide you with the resilience to participate in social activities with your friends and family. How can you stay socially active? A great way to do this is to plan your activities yourself and in sufficient detail. If you want to go to dinner and a movie, then you reserve your energy during the day, so you can go out in the evening. I use this tactic a lot. If I have a late meeting, then I start my day later and conserve my energy in the day so that it's available for me in the evening. If my husband wants to go out for dinner and a movie, I take a short nap that afternoon to help my body recharge and be ready for the evening.

You can do this too! These are tried and true tips and I know they will work for you.

CHAPTER 6

WHY IS GOD MAD AT ME?

I don't want to say that I "grew up in church" but my sister and I would go to church every Sunday. There was a church bus that would drive around the neighborhood on Sunday mornings and pick up people to go to Sunday school. My parents didn't take us to church and my sister and I wanted to go, so we would get up early every Sunday morning.

The church was considered to be a Southern Baptist denomination. I can remember that the preacher would continue to preach until someone walked up the aisle and accepted Christ into their life. Sometimes the sermon would last over an hour until someone felt the spirit of

Christ sweep over them and they walked up that aisle.

I don't remember what led up to my decision to walk up that aisle. I don't remember if I went first or if my sister did. But, in the fall of 1977, my sister and I walked up that aisle. This meant that both of us had decided to live Christian lives. I was eleven and my sister was seventeen.

In the true spirit of a Southern Baptist church, there was a baptismal pool in the sanctuary. When the Preacher decided there were enough people to baptize, the oval-shaped baptismal pool would be filled with about 125 gallons of water and those being baptized would don white robes, walk up the three or four steps to the pool, step into the water, and be fully immersed by the preacher. For whatever reason, I went into the water before my sister, thus making me the first one in my family to be baptized.

I wasn't afraid to be baptized. I remember feeling a sense of calm about the entire experience. Other than my sister, none of my family members were present. I don't remember why my parents chose not to go; I had an older sister and an older brother who were married and living their own lives, so I didn't count on them being there.

My choice to believe in a higher power has helped me through some very tough times in my life. I would often turn to prayer whenever I was faced with difficult life decisions or when I felt slighted by someone that I thought was a friend.

But living every day in pain has me asking the same questions over and over: Why me? Why do I have to suffer every day in pain? Why was I taken away from my career as a nurse practitioner? Why have I been forced to change everything about my life? What did I do to deserve this?

My educated brain tells me that questions such as these are ridiculous. There is no force conspiring against me, but part of me still thinks that I'm being punished for something.

Some people, when faced with tragedy, discard their faith and their beliefs. Others are just the opposite: their faith and belief become stronger. Then there are others who fall in the middle: they deny their faith when life is particularly bad (e.g., *if there is a God, he wouldn't let this happen to me*) and they revel in their faith when life is going great (e.g., *God must really be on my side because it doesn't get any better than this*).

Two years ago, a very dear friend of my family was killed in a motorcycle accident. He was my oldest son's best friend and best man at his wedding. He practically grew up in my home.

While he was driving home from work on Halloween, he was hit by a car and was killed instantly. This young man was a very staunch believer in God and was truly a disciple of Christ.

He didn't drink, and he didn't smoke. He was honest, caring, and loving. He would give you the shirt off his back. I still think about him every day. And I still wonder why he was taken away so soon.

My Christian upbringing tells me not to question occurrences such as this because it is "all part of God's plan." Just like it is part of God's plan to have me in my current predicament.

As a healthcare provider, I want to understand everything at a scientific level, so it causes much inner turmoil when I am forced to "just accept things." My spiritual being is very curious and inquisitive. I definitely haven't lost faith, but my faith hasn't gotten any stronger since I've been faced with the daily challenge of a life in pain.

I have learned to take life day-by-day and sometimes minute-by-minute. I frequently remind myself that on days when my pain is unbearable, it is only temporary and that I'm not going to feel the same tomorrow morning.

Living every day with pain can be depressing to say the least. There have been times when I have gone to bed at night and didn't care if I woke up the next morning or not.

There have also been times when I have thought that my family would be better off without me. I don't have these thoughts every day. I have them on days when my pain level is at its worst.

According to Lipka and Gecewicz,[20] 27 percent of adults in the U.S. consider themselves spiritual but not religious. This number is up 8 percent over the past five years. A study by Büssing, Reiser, Michalsen Zahn, and Baumann[21] found that 56 percent of patients with a chronic disease believed in a guardian angel "often" or "regularly." Even more interesting was that 38 percent of those people did not identify themselves as religious or spiritual. People may use this belief to try to make sense out of their daily struggle to manage their pain.

---

[20] Lipka, M. & Gecewicz, C. (2017). More Americans say they're spiritual but not religious. Retrieved from:
http://www.pewresearch.org/fact-tank/2017/09/06/more-americans-now-say-theyre-spiritual-but-not-religious/
[21] Büssing A., Reiser F., Michalsen A., Zahn A., and Baumann K. (2015). Do patients with chronic pain diseases believe in guardian angels: Even in a secular society? A cross-sectional study among German patients with chronic diseases. *Journal of Religious Health*, 76-86. DOI: 10.1007/s10943-013-9735-9.

There are several studies[22,23] documenting the positive effects of prayer on chronic pain. There have even been studies evaluating if active prayer is more effective than passive prayer. There are even specific prayers that can be said that are supposed to make your pain go away. There are prayers for chronic pain, prayers for friends who are in pain, and prayers for accepting help.

Suicide is the tenth leading cause of death in the United States and 44,000 Americans die by suicide each year. There is one death by suicide for every twenty-five attempts. Suicide rates are highest among adults between forty-five and sixty-four at 19.6 percent. The second highest rate is 19.4 among those eighty-five years or older.[24]

These numbers are alarming, yet there is still a taboo surrounding suicidal thoughts. You tell someone that you've had suicidal thoughts and they immediately think that there is a lot more wrong with you than your chronic pain. Why

---

[22] Chitterjan, A., & Rajiv, R. (2009). Prayer and healing: A medical and scientific perspective on randomized controlled trials. *Indian Journal of Psychiatry, (51)*, 247-253. DOI: 10.4103/0019-5545.58288
[23] Science proves the healing power of prayer. (31 March 2015). Retrieved from https://www.newsmax.com/health/headline/prayer-health-faith-medicine/2015/03/31/id/635623/
[24] http://www.mentalhealthamerica.net/suicide

can't we just be honest with these thoughts? Why can't I tell someone that dealing with pain every day makes me question if my life has any value?

I started seeing a counselor about six months ago at the urging of my pain doctor. I remember telling my pain doctor, "I don't know how I can put up with this pain for the rest of my life." This statement was enough for my doctor to think I was suicidal.

In the beginning, I would see my counselor every week. At that first visit, she asked me very direct questions about my thoughts concerning my pain. Such directness made me feel very uncomfortable. I had never been asked questions that got directly to the heart of the matter. This was new to me.

My counselor has helped me learn how to challenge my negative thoughts. My spirituality has helped me overcome these negative thoughts.

It's important to point out that spirituality isn't religion. Spirituality includes your soul, your hopes, your beliefs, and your emotions. Some people may discover that their spiritual life is intricately linked to their association with a church, temple, mosque, or synagogue; others may pray or find reassurance in a personal relationship with God or a higher power; still others seek meaning through their connections to nature or art. Like your sense of purpose, your personal definition of spirituality may change throughout your life, adapting to your own experiences and relationships.

Call to Action

Ask yourself if you are religious or spiritual or both. Turn to your faith leader, minister, priest, preacher, etc., and tell them how you feel. Ask for their prayers and guidance. Pray for yourself or someone you care about.

Studies show that individuals rely on their spirituality and religious faith when coping with illness, and that these religious and spiritual forms of coping are generally associated with positive health outcomes, including less depression.[25] Spirituality and activities can lessen the presence or severity of pain by improving your mood. Religious and spiritual beliefs have also been linked with general happiness and life satisfaction. In addition, people who reported strong religious and/or spiritual beliefs had a reduced sensitivity to pain.[22]

---

[25] Wachholtz, A.B., Pearce, M.J. & Koenig, H. (2007). *Journal of Behavioral Medicine*. 30: 311. https://doi.org/10.1007/s10865-007-9114-7

CHAPTER 7

SHOW ME THE MONEY

I consider myself fortunate to have the job that I do. I am a college professor for graduate nursing students. I always wanted to end my nursing career in education, but I thought I would be older when I went this direction.

As a nurse, my pain became more excruciating, and I needed more and more medication just to get through the day. I would take high doses of Prednisone, a medication that helps with inflammation and swelling.

It made me feel great! My pain was tolerable, I had a lot of energy and I was able to think clearly. But taking high doses of Prednisone isn't without side effects.

On average, I was taking 60 mg of Prednisone a day. This high dose caused me to gain seventy pounds which was terrible for my chronic pain, not to mention the other problems associated with obesity.

I realized that managing my chronic pain with Prednisone and a stressful job were not conducive to good health. So, I went on the job hunt and two years ago I took a job at a small, private Catholic college in Columbus, Ohio.

I am the Coordinator of the Nurse Practitioner programs and an Associate Professor. Having worked in intensive care units as a nurse practitioner for the majority of my life, going to work in a college took a little getting used to. My work hours are 9:00 a.m.–5:00 p.m. Monday through Friday. As a nurse, I worked ten- or twelve-hour days three to four days a week. The pace is much slower and job-related stress is practically non-existent when compared to my prior working environment.

Having a better work environment has allowed me to focus on my health. I've lost the seventy pounds I gained from steroids and I have more peace of mind.

One of the best parts of my job is the flexibility. The majority of my job can be done any place where I have a computer and access to the Internet. This means that if I'm having a rough day because of pain, I can work from home.

As a Nurse Practitioner who was managing the ills of several patients a day, working from home was not an option. And nursing is the only profession I know of where the higher your education, the less money you make.

Having a doctorate degree is a customary qualification needed for a career in higher education and it was a required qualification for my current job. However, getting my doctorate degree did nothing for my Nurse Practitioner career—I didn't earn more money or take on additional responsibility. Obtaining my doctorate was just something that I did many years ago because I wanted to.

When I changed jobs and started working at the college, my pay also changed—and not for the better. I took a significant pay cut and, because I had a new employer, I had to change my health insurance. The change in health insurance meant that I had to find new physicians who would accept my insurance.

My pain physician, who has been treating me for years, is considered out-of-network. This means that my insurance company has negotiated lower payments to specific pain physicians for treating patients.

I didn't want to find a new physician who

wasn't familiar with me and all my previous medical history and procedures. I also didn't want to try to explain all of it to someone new.

It takes a long time to explain to someone all of the MRIs, CT scans, X-rays, injections, physical therapy, warm water therapy, acupuncture, all the non-steroidal anti-inflammatory medicines I've tried (which is all of them), how many times I've had radiofrequency nerve root ablation, etc. The list goes on!

Even if you send a new physician all those records, many of them will ask you if you'll "go through it" with them. Really? We'll be here for hours!

So, going to someone new isn't an option; I chose to keep my current pain physician who is out-of-network and costs me $150 out-of-pocket every four weeks. That's just for my visit and doesn't include any medications, injections, compounded creams, or patches.

One day, one of the nurses in the office suggested that we call my insurance company and ask them for an allowance to continue to see my pain physician but at the in-network price. The process took about three months to complete, but eventually my insurance company agreed to discount the price of my monthly visits. This has saved—and will continue to save—me a lot of money.

The cost of chronic pain isn't cheap. I have never stopped to calculate the personal cost to me—I'm afraid to know the actual number. Between the decrease in pay, the out-of-pocket expenses for physicians and mental health counselors, the cost of medications, and lost productivity at work, I know that it's a lot of money.

In a working paper published by the National Bureau of Economic Research[26] researchers found that Americans over the age of fifty with chronic pain are so unhappy that they'd need to earn between $20,000 and $50,000 per year more to be as happy as they would be otherwise with no pain.

Another way of looking at it: People would pay between $56 and $145 per day to be just as happy as they otherwise are, but pain-free.[27] Researchers think this data will be important to policymakers, so the policymaker will get an idea of how much financial resources should be allotted to treat pain.

Billions of dollars are spent each year on the treatment of chronic pain. In a 2011 study by Johns Hopkins University and George Washington University, researchers found that if

---

[26] http://www.nber.org/
[27] https://www.vox.com/policy-and-politics/2017/8/10/16118620/how-much-is-pain-worth

you combine the health care costs to treat pain with lost productivity from people missing days at work, chronic pain costs the United States health care system between $560 billion and $635 billion per year. This is much more than the cost of cancer, diabetes, or heart disease.[25]

However, according to Institute of Medicine Committee on Advancing Pain Research, Care, and Education (2011) the $560–635 billion range is a conservative estimate because it excludes the cost of pain affecting institutionalized individuals (including nursing home residents and corrections inmates), military personnel, children under age eighteen, and personal caregivers (such as spouses who miss work while caring for people with pain), as well as the lost productivity of workers younger than twenty-four and older than sixty-five. The estimate also excludes the emotional cost of pain.

The emotional cost of pain can lead to decreased social interactions, diminished leisure activities and a reduction in social contacts. In addition, a study in Canada noted that half of the patients in pain indicated that their condition had prevented them from attending social or family events (Moulin, et al., 2002).

It may become difficult for the pain sufferer to continue working because of the severity of their pain. In addition, their employer may have provided their health insurance—without their employer, health insurance is more expensive and has higher deductibles. With limitations on earning a living, and the uncertainty of finding affordable health insurance, there can be significant changes in access to physicians, food, and shelter.

Disability is an option for some, but disability payments are usually just a fraction of what you were earning when working full-time. In addition, the process of applying for disability can be lengthy and cumbersome. You may deplete your savings or even lose your home. I've seen couples divorce because of the stress associated with their uncertain financial future. Being reckless with your money is going to negatively affect your partner and the overall longevity of your relationship.[28]

Living with chronic pain is very costly. There may be hospital bills, doctor visits, the cost of medications, the time and expense of traveling, mental health counseling, the cost of assistive devices such as wheelchairs, canes, and maybe even a special bed, and even potentially needing to hire someone to do things like

---

[28] Myers, S. (2012). How financial problems & stress cause divorce. *Psychology Today*. Retrieved from https://www.psychologytoday.com/blog/insight-is-2020/201212/how-financial-problems-stress-cause-divorce

cleaning your house.

You will need to change some aspects of your life to appropriately plan for the financial impact of pain. Just as you have changed parts of your lifestyle, you will also have to change parts of your budget.

Call to Action

So how can you and your family manage the financial manifestations of chronic pain? For people who were working when pain came into their life, they probably experienced (like I did) a shift in social status and a change to their lifestyle.

One way to plan for the financial impact of chronic pain is by planning ahead. You can plan ahead by contacting a financial planner. A financial planner can help you get your finances in order so that you will be financially sound in the future. A financial planner can also tell you how much money you need to save and how to invest your money so that you are prepared for retirement. The financial planner can help you figure out what type of investments you need to make and what type of mortgage is best for your situation. Other benefits of having a financial planner include: how much money to keep in your emergency fund, what type and how much insurance you need, and how and when to downsize.

It is also a good idea to set up a realistic budget. There are numerous websites that can help you set up a budget for free. You can find this information in the resources section. By creating a budget, you can pay down your bills in a timely manner, safeguard your credit, and plan for future expenses. This is very helpful if you have a progressive physical condition, so that you can make sure you will have enough money in the future.

Additionally, it is a good idea to continue to work as long as physically possible. You may need to modify your work environment or revise your job description. By working as long as physically possible, this will provide an additional layer of financial safety for when the time comes and you are no longer able to work due to chronic pain.

You may need to ask for accommodations at work so that you can work comfortably. For example, if you have a job that requires a lot of sitting, an ergonomically designed chair may be the difference between working or not.

You could also ask to shift your work time. For example, if mornings are difficult for you, instead of working from 9:00 a.m. to 5:00 p.m., you could work from 10:00 a.m. to 6:00 p.m.

Or maybe you need a longer lunch break, so you can take a "power nap." A short, twenty-minute nap can boost your mood and productivity. There are several companies that have nap rooms to encourage these power naps!

For me, being able to work from home has increased my productivity immensely. I can work in blocks of time—three or four hours at a time—and then take a short break. On those mornings where I can't sleep, I'll start my work day at 4:00 a.m. Other days, I'll start my day at 7:00 a.m. Being able to continue to work can improve your outlook on life and mental health.

Another way to tackle the financial problems of chronic pain, is to live frugally. For example, it is usually cheaper to buy your meat in bulk. I buy ground beef in five-pound packages. Then, when I get home, I divide it up into one-pound packages, put it in a freezer-safe plastic bag, and freeze it until I need it. Or you can buy a whole ham at the grocery store and ask the deli to slice it. This is a cheaper way to have sandwich meat.

One way that I help cut costs in my family is to grow fresh vegetables. I have several elevated garden troughs on my deck and every year I grow tomatoes, peppers, and various other vegetables so that I can preserve them and make soups out of them for the winter. Fresh vegetables always taste better than store-bought ones and I don't have to worry about what kinds of pesticides or insecticides have been put on the vegetables. You can even pick your own fruits and vegetables at local farms. To find a local farm in your area that allows you to pick your own, you can visit www.pickyourown.org.

Are you an impulse buyer? Instead of carrying credit cards, carry cash. When you actually see the money disappearing, you'll think twice about that purchase. Another way to curb impulse buying is to ask yourself why you're shopping in the first place. Are you shopping just to cheer yourself up? Take a walk or call a friend. Walking and talking are free and you won't be shocked by a high credit card bill arriving in the mail.

Small changes can have big results. For additional tips on living frugally, visit the website livingfrugaltips.com.

CHAPTER 8

TYPHOID JILL

In my prior life (before chronic pain) I belonged to an organization called the Ohio Disaster Medical Assistance Team, or OH-5 DMAT.

During emergencies, disasters, and large-scale national security events, a DMAT may be deployed to the area to assist people in the event medical treatment is needed. A Disaster Medical Assistance Team consists of medical personnel and supplies, communication personnel and supplies, logistics experts, and administrative personnel. The organization is voluntary but, if you are training or on a deployment, you are paid.

I was a member of the Ohio DMAT for eleven years. I joined in 2002 shortly after the events of

9/11. As a former firefighter and paramedic, I was deeply moved by the tragedy that struck the people of New York and Washington, and my sense of public service was awakened once again.

While a member of the DMAT, I was deployed to national political conventions and too many hurricanes to count. I spent several weeks in Mississippi on two different deployments during Hurricane Katrina and wouldn't trade my experiences for anything. I found the people of Biloxi, Mississippi to be very friendly and appreciative toward the members of my DMAT.

I was also pre-deployed to Atlanta, GA after the Haiti earthquake in 2010. It was then that I believe my pain problems began.

The Haitian earthquake in January 2010 registered 7.0 on the Richter scale and was followed by two aftershocks that registered 5.9 and 5.5. It was estimated that three million people were affected by the quake—nearly one-third of the country's total population. Of these, over one million were left homeless in the immediate aftermath.[29]

Due to the widespread devastation, the basic infrastructure was absent. This meant unsanitary conditions, lack of fresh water, and

---

[29] https://www.britannica.com/event/Haiti-earthquake-of-2010

hospitals that were left in crumbled heaps.

Prior to being deployed, all members of DMAT had to receive the typhoid vaccine. I received my vaccine at a Travel and Immunization Center in Columbus, Ohio.

I can't remember the exact timeline—if it was twenty-four or thirty-six hours—but I woke up in the pre-dawn hours of the day I was supposed to fly to Atlanta. Our team was going to be pre-staged in Atlanta, Georgia. This meant that we would wait in Atlanta until military transportation was arranged for us to fly to Haiti.

I woke up shivering uncontrollably. I felt cold all the way down to my bones. I didn't think too much of it at the time; it was January and my husband liked to keep our bedroom cool.

I thought that a hot shower would help me warm up. The shower felt great. The water was very warm, and the bathroom was all steamed up. But when I got out of the shower, the uncontrollable shivering started again. I was shivering so violently that I couldn't even get dressed.

Now I started wondering what was going on.

I woke up my husband—who is a human furnace—cuddled up next to him underneath several blankets, and tried to warm up. I fell back to sleep for another forty-five minutes until it was time to go to the airport.

I was scheduled to fly out of the Dayton Airport, which was seventy miles away from my home in Columbus. My husband loaded my bags into the car and we took off for the airport.

The trip from Columbus to Dayton was more of an adventure than a simple drive to the airport. I felt awful. I was sick to my stomach and freezing. I thought it was just nerves. I'd never been to an area that had been devastated by an earthquake and I was definitely nervous.

We had to stop the car and pullover at least three times on the way to the airport because I was throwing up so much, although at that point I didn't have anything in my stomach so I was just dry-heaving.

As a woman in my forties who had born children, sometimes when you violently gag, you leak a little pee. Well, this happened to me too. Every time we stopped on the side of the interstate, I would dry heave and wet my pants. I thought if I could just make it to the airport, I could get another pair of pants and undies out of my bag and I'd be okay.

Wouldn't you know it, my commanding officer was standing at the main entrance to the airport on the watch for all of his DMAT members. Adjusting my previous plan, I tied my jacket around my waist, complained that I was warm and needed to take my jacket off, and I casually walked to the bathroom.

Once I was in the bathroom, I changed clothes, put my wet clothes in a plastic bag that I had packed, and met up with the rest of my team members.

The flight from Dayton to Atlanta is less than an hour and since the flight was so short, dining service was not offered, nor was it available. As soon as the plane took off, my nausea and queasiness came back. The flight attendant sat me in the first row so I could be close to the lavatory. I asked for saltines or a Sprite or 7-Up, only to be told that the plane carried neither. I was given an emesis bag and a glass of water.

I began to accept the fact that this wasn't nerves. I was sick. I was sick like I'd never been sick in my life. I was having some bizarre reaction to the typhoid vaccine and I was stuck on a plane. I just wanted to curl up under a mound of blankets and sleep for a week or two.

I don't remember landing. I don't remember how we got to our hotel. I just remember being in my hotel bathroom, sitting on the toilet with the trashcan in front of me. The next thing I remember was looking out of my hotel room and seeing my team members getting on a bus to be driven to the Atlanta airport on their way to Haiti. Later, someone left a plain bagel outside of my door.

I wasn't able to go to Haiti because I was quarantined in my hotel room until I was able to keep food down. I don't remember the plane ride home or my husband driving me home from the airport.

In hindsight, I now realize that those few days were only the beginning of my troubles. After I returned from Atlanta, I went back to my job as a Nurse Practitioner and went about my life . . . until I started having severe back pain.

I went to my family physician, who referred me to a neurosurgeon, who performed a thorough exam and non-invasive imaging. The diagnosis was nonspecific, meaning that there wasn't an exact cause of the pain—no obviously ruptured disc and no fractures in my vertebrae.

I endured several rounds of physical therapy which included aqua therapy (exercising in very warm water to relieve pressure on your joints), specific exercises to strengthen my core and lower back, heat therapy, massage therapy, etc. You name it and I tried it. Nothing worked. My pain was still intense and was starting to interfere with my life.

I continued to see my family physician with complaints of low back pain. The pain was getting worse and I was having trouble sleeping. I tried every over-the-counter treatment that I could think of: heating pads, ice packs, non-steroidal anti-inflammatory medicines, aspirin, pain patches, massage therapy, aromatherapy, acupuncture, and relaxation techniques. If someone would have told me to stand on my head and whistle with a mouth full of peanut butter and my pain would be better, I would have tried it. In other words, I was desperate.

Several months passed. I was getting frustrated and my family physician was getting frustrated. Nothing he prescribed for my pain was working. So my family physician referred me to a pain specialist.

The first pain specialist I went to was not a good fit for me. He walked in the exam room, stared at my chart, and said I needed a spinal stimulator. He didn't do a physical exam. He didn't check my range of motion. He didn't even say hello to me.

I was stunned. As a healthcare provider, I would never have treated a patient so badly, so nonchalantly. I must have looked at the doctor in an odd way, because he then asked, "Didn't you watch the video?"

I said, "No, what video?"

He yelled at me and said, "If you're not going to help yourself, how do you expect me to?" He then stormed out of the room.

I just sat there. I couldn't believe what had

just happened. I left his office, went out to my car, and started crying. I called my husband and explained to him what had happened in the doctor's office.

Thankfully, my husband is a very reasonable man. His calm demeanor and my heated demeanor balance each other out. But, on that day, my husband asked me if I would like to go back in there and tell the doctor how I felt.

I, of course, said "Yes."

So, I got out of my car and walked back into the doctor's office. The waiting room was full of patients, but that didn't deter me. I went to the receptionist's desk and said, "I want to speak to the doctor." I was told that he was in an exam room with another patient, so I decided to tell the receptionist—and everyone in the waiting room—my opinion of the doctor's "bedside manner."

I was pretty angry and probably lucky that the police weren't called because I was ranting and raving like a lunatic. But I did get my point across and I did file a complaint with the Ohio Board of Medicine for the way that I was treated.

This episode was an eye-opener. I suddenly understood that my life had changed. Who I identified as had also changed. I was going to be looked at different and treated differently because now I was a woman with chronic pain.

I told my family physician about the incident at the pain doctor's office. My family physician referred me to another pain specialist. This time I was lucky. I found a pain doctor who truly cared about me and my pain. That was several years ago—I still see the same pain doctor every four weeks like clockwork.

I eventually had a spinal stimulator implanted. A spinal cord stimulator directs mild electrical pulses to interfere with pain messages reaching the brain. A small device implanted near the spine generates these pulses.[30] The battery-powered generator is about the size of a pacemaker and is implanted near my left hip.

For me, the stimulator takes the edge off the pain. I keep it on about eighteen hours a day and I charge it about once a week. I hate charging because I'm limited in what I can do while charging.

My life revolves around my visits to my pain doctor and charging my stimulator. Life isn't as carefree or spontaneous as it used to be—this is my onus to bear. Vacations and business trips are planned around these facets of my life.

One could argue that this really isn't pain control; I'm still controlled by doctor visits,

---

[30] www.spinehealth.com

medications, and the need for electricity to keep my stimulator charged. However, it's the best strategy that I have, so I roll with it.

Over the past two years I have also come to the realization that I may not be able to work as long as I had once hoped. This is detrimental to my psyche because for me, work is my hobby. I've always worked two or three jobs at a time, but I'm beginning to realize that this may not be possible in the future because my daily regimen can be very tiring.

Several months ago, I started seeing a therapist to help me manage my internal thoughts about my quality of life. At times, I have very dark thoughts about not being able to the things that I used to do and not being able to do the things that I want to do.

While performing research for this book, I found several studies describing how chronic pain impacts quality of life. As a person who is based in science, I found this comforting. I knew that my quality of life was very different that before, but it was nice to know that I wasn't alone.

Research by Lamé, Peters, Vlaeyen, Kleef, and Patijan[31] found that patients with chronic

---

[31] Lamé, I.E., Peters, M.L., Vlaeyen, J.W., Kleef, M.V., & Patijn, J. (2005). Quality of life in chronic pain is more associated with

pain experience a very low quality of life. They also found that patients with low back pain and patients with multiple pain locations have the lowest quality of life. Women reported more pain and more depressive thoughts about pain. Women also reported more disability and poorer quality of life. I'm not surprised by this. At times, I think that women do not receive the same level of care as men. This leads to their pain being less controlled, which in turn leads to depression and poor quality of life.

Breivik, Collett, Ventafridda, Cohen, and Gallacher[32] called over 46,000 patients with chronic pain and asked them about their experiences. Many patients reported a pain intensity of ≥5 on a 10-point Numeric Rating Scale (NRS) during their last episode of pain. In-depth interviews also showed that 21 percent had been diagnosed with depression because of their pain, 61 percent were less able or unable to work outside the home, 19 percent had lost their job and 13 percent had changed jobs because of their pain.

---

beliefs about pain, than with pain intensity. *European Journal of Pain, 9,* 15-24. DOI: 10.1016/j.ejpain.2004.02.006

[32] Breivik, H., Collett, B., Ventafridda, V., Cohen, R., Gallacher, D. (2006). Survey of chronic pain in Europe: prevalence, impact on daily life, and treatment. *European Journal of Pain, 10,* 287-333. DOI: 10.1016/j.ejpain.2005.06.009

I'm sure many of you can relate to these statistics. Your pain isn't at an acceptable level, you feel depressed, and you've had to change how much you work or where you work. I know that I have experienced all of this because of my chronic pain.

As a Nurse Practitioner, I think that these statistics are unacceptable. As a chronic pain patient, I *know* they are unacceptable.

I want to continue to work and be a contributing member of society. Keeping your mind and body moving is beneficial for your mental, physical, and financial health.

We all want to feel needed and we all want to make a lasting impression in life. Living with chronic pain impacts different people in various ways. Some people with chronic pain may never stop working; others find that their condition interrupts their career; and still others may be able to do only limited work. Some people with chronic pain find that they are able, with minor accommodations, to work in the same way they did before. Others may have to re-enter work gradually.

You may encounter roadblocks and setbacks due to your chronic pain, but remember: contributing to something that is meaningful to you can bring you a sense of purpose. Meaningful activity enhances your self-esteem by improving your skills and helping you accomplish your personal goals and feel good about yourself. Meaningful activity can include school, volunteer work, part-time work, and full-time employment, and also enables you to meet new people and make friends. All of this can improve the quality of your life.

What are some ways that you can improve your quality of life? One way is to find products that make your home environment more comfortable. For example, getting a good night's sleep has been shown to improve your pain level and thus, your quality of life. There are several different types of pillows, shapes of pillows, and stuffing of pillows that can help you sleep better. You can also add a layer of foam or even a feather-top mattress cover to your bed. This can also enhance your sleep.

You can also be sure that you have appropriate aids to make your daily activities such as showering, easier to do. You could put a shower seat in your shower, so you can sit down while sudsing. You should also have a non-slip bath mat in your shower, so you won't fall. These are just a couple of ideas to improve your quality of life.

WHAT NEXT?

In writing this book, I wanted to let other chronic pain sufferers know that they are not alone. I wanted to assure others who, like me, have suffered in silence, too afraid to ask for help, too afraid to tell our healthcare provider how bad we really feel for fear that we would be labeled as lazy or as an addict.

We're not lazy. We're not addicts looking for our next high. We're not making up our symptoms to get sympathy from people. We're people who have been given a life sentence. Chronic pain is a thief. It steals time, relationships, independence, spontaneity, and hope. Millions of people suffer from chronic pain and all the consequences that go along with it.

My hope is that you have learned much and been comforted more after reading this book. I hope that you have learned that there are millions of people just like you who are living with pain every day. We, just like you, plan on what activities we will do each day for each hour and sometimes for each and every minute.

My hope is that by reading some of my personal stories—whether challenging, embarrassing, or inspirational—you can identify with a small part of them.

Have you had to cancel a commitment at the last minute because your bucket of steps was empty? I have.

Have you lashed out at someone in frustration or anger because you've been in pain all day? I have.

Have you thought that you were a burden to your family and that they would be better off without you? I have.

Have you given up your dream because of your pain? Have you changed where you work or how many hours you work? I have.

Has your pain dictated the type of car you drive or the kind of clothes you wear? Mine has.

Chronic pain doesn't have to dominate every facet of my life or yours! We can *Survive and Thrive* with chronic pain. We can discover how to earmark our steps throughout the day, so we don't have to cancel commitments at the last minute.

We can stretch, use heating pads, ice packs, grabbers, and any other piece of equipment that is going to help us get through our day easier.

We can confront our emotions. We can tell our "team members" how we feel without fear of repercussions. They can cheer us on, accept us for who we are, and be there to support us through thick and thin.

We can deny that our pain is here to stay. We can grieve the loss of what once was. We can get angry and try to bargain our way out of being in chronic pain.

After we have worked through the denial, grief, and anger, we will turn the corner and start to recognize rational solutions to our daily challenges. And then we will start to accept our new "normal" and allow ourselves to hope and dream about our future as a person with chronic pain who is not only surviving but *thriving* with chronic pain.

By reading this book, I hope you realize that you are not alone. There are millions of us who suffer from chronic pain. We are resilient, and we will give 100 percent to everything we do, minute-by-minute and day-by-day.

ARE YOU READY TO
TAKE CONTROL OF YOUR LIFE OVER
CHRONIC PAIN?

I would love to help you. For more
information, please visit my website:
www.drjbkirby.com

ABOUT THE AUTHOR

As a Nurse Practitioner with over 30 years of experience in healthcare, Dr. JB Kirby has seen it all including deployments to natural disasters with the Department of Homeland Security.

After spending most of her career at the bedside, she was sidelined with a rare pain disorder called Adhesive Arachnoiditis. In 2015, she decided to reclaim control of her life from suffering and she is now a Pain Coach and College Professor.

Dr. Kirby has lectured at national and international conferences during her time as a Nurse Practitioner about ways to survive and thrive with such devastating illnesses as cancer and debilitating pain disorders. She has been on Capitol Hill in Washington D.C. to counsel lawmakers concerning pain management and the opioid crisis. Her expertise in the field of pain study and management is only surpassed by her willingness to discuss and mentor others who have the same feelings of desperation and despair she experiences waking up each morning with chronic pain.

Yes, Dr. Kirby has seen it all, done it all and, unfortunately, felt it all. She knows all about the, "Why Me?" syndrome a person goes through during the darkest hours when the suffering seems as if it will never end. She can hold your hand and lead you through those times and show you that there is a way to live your life to the fullest. Dr. Kirby is married with 3 sons. She lives in Columbus, Ohio with her husband and 4 fur babies.

Now that you've read my book, please go to Amazon and leave an honest review. I look forward to hearing your thoughts!

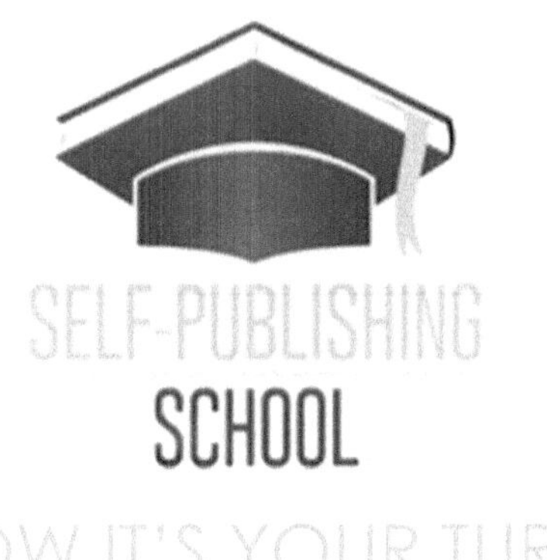

Discover the EXACT 3-step blueprint you need to become a bestselling author in 3 months.

Self-Publishing School helped me, and now I want them to help you with this FREE WEBINAR!

Even if you're busy, bad at writing, or don't know where to start, you CAN write a bestseller and build your best life.

With tools and experience across a variety niches and professions, Self-Publishing School is the <u>only</u> resource you need to take your book to the finish line!

DON'T WAIT
Watch this FREE WEBINAR now, and
Say "YES" to becoming a bestseller:
https://xe172.isrefer.com/go/sps4fta-vts/bookbrosinc4361